BEET
the
ODDS

Harness the Power of Beets to
Radically Transform Your Health

Nathan S. Bryan, PhD
Carolyn Pierini CLS (ASCP), CNC

Neogenis Laboratories
248 Addie Roy Rd Suite #B201
Austin, TX 78746
www.neogenis.com

Printed in the United States of America.

The information in this book is for educational purposes only. It is not intended to replace the advice of a physician or medical practitioner. Please consult your healthcare provider before beginning any new health program.

ISBN 978-1-9888135-0-2

10 9 8 7 6 5 4 3 2

Nathan S. Bryan, PhD is an Assistant Professor of Molecular Medicine within the Brown Foundation Institute of Molecular Medicine, part of the School of Medicine at the University of Texas Health Science Center at Houston. He is also on faculty within the Department of Integrative Biology and Pharmacology and Graduate School of Biomedical Sciences at the UT Houston Medical School. Dr. Bryan earned his undergraduate Bachelor of Science degree in Biochemistry from the University of Texas at Austin and his doctoral degree from Louisiana State University School of Medicine in Shreveport where he was the recipient of the Dean's Award for Excellence in Research. He pursued his post-doctoral training as a Kirschstein Fellow at Boston University School of Medicine in the Whitaker Cardiovascular Institute. Dr. Bryan joined the Institute of Molecular Medicine, University of Texas Health Science Center in Houston, in June 2006. Dr. Bryan's research is dedicated to providing a better understanding of the key role nitric oxide plays in health and disease. He devoted 12 years of research into diagnosing nitric oxide (N-O) insufficiency and natural strategies to restore N-O production in the body. What was discovered may provide the basis for new preventive and therapeutic strategies in diseases associated with N-O insufficiency and new fundamental guidelines for optimal health.

Dr. Bryan has published a number of highly cited papers and authored or edited 4 books.

Carolyn Pierini CLS (ASCP), CNC is a (California-licensed) Clinical Laboratory Scientist and Medical Microbiologist with over 20 years experience in the hospital laboratory departments of chemistry, hematology, immunology, and in particular, microbiology. The effects of nutrient growth factors on microbial morphology eventually led her to the biochemistry of human nutrigenomics - an area of functional medicine that identifies the effects of food, lifestyle and environmental factors as major determinants for the state of one's health.

As a nutritional consultant, Carolyn began educating others about the epigenetic science of achieving optimal health, incorporating innovative approaches and using routine blood and urine chemistry findings for identifying patterns related to nutritional needs. She has authored numerous technical articles and professional materials for health care providers, has been a technical advisor to doctors, educational webinar host, TV and radio guest panelist, lecturer and formulation consultant. Investigating underlying causes for disease naturally led her into nitric oxide education because of its primary, foundational significance in human health.

*Vegetables and fruits
contain the anti-carcinogenic cocktail
to which we are adapted.
We abandon it at our peril.*

Epidemiologist, John Potter MD

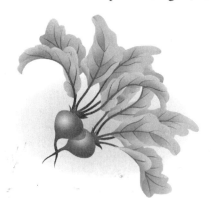

Contents

Introduction

How is it possible that we missed this? Our ancestors didn't miss it. How could we have ignored a food that has been faithfully passed to us through countless generations - a food whose appearance is the clue that shouts to us – the one food that possesses the extraordinary benefit for our own heart and circulatory system? It's just a mere oversight that nearly cost us our lives, as heart disease is the number one killer of humans. But the truth is about to set us free.

Re-welcome, *Beta vulgaris* or beetroot (beet, table, red or garden beet), a truly remarkable food gift to the human body that is now getting the attention it deserves. After all, from leaves to root this vegetable has sustained many civilizations for thousands of years. Beet leaves are undoubtedly nutritious and tasty but it is the beet root that will be the central focus of this book. The beloved beet plant has survived through cultivation to the present because of one simple but important fact – *extreme nutritional value*.

The beet appeared to have lost its popularity in some places but remained a traditional mainstay in others such as in Eastern and Central Europe and India. Some speculate that beets were usurped by spinach. The good news is that the beleaguered beet is making a triumphant comeback thanks to science and a greater understanding of the power contained within it. If someone does not become a disciple of beets through taste, at least initially, they just might come around once they discover the miraculous health benefits that beets can provide.

Perhaps the most under-appreciated food in the history of eating is the beet. Historically, as a source of food, it was easily grown most of the year, had long storability and adapted well to a wide variety of climates. From the earliest times of medicine, beets have been used to address:

- kidney dysfunction

- skin and dandruff complaints

- fever

- heart disease

- anemia and blood disorders

- poor circulation

- cancer

- liver and gallbladder conditions

- constipation

- alertness and energy needs

- sexual performance

Today, the beet is still used as a "functional" food to support a wide range of health concerns and beet powder is an active ingredient in multiple types of nutritional supplements. However, beets and beet powders can vary significantly in their effectiveness.

Beet science is found in medical literature with published clinical studies examining important constituents in the beet that impact human physiology. The most popular studies focus on the beet's ability to help boost stamina, improve cognition through enhanced blood flow to the brain, and support heart health. Beets contain familiar vitamins and minerals but also unique plant or "phyto" nutrients which are often referred to as phytochemicals. These powerful substances can "speak" or convey a message to the cell's genes (DNA) directing them to make other crucial compounds that support and protect the body.

Beets have become the "edge" in competitive elite sport and were recently consumed by some athletes in the 2012 Olympic Games improving their performance by as much as 16%. This fact alone has piqued serious interest in beets.

This book is a simple but comprehensive look at the remarkable value of beets. It moves through supporting facts to climax with the discovery of the most significant beet benefit in all of its history. Harnessing the power hidden in the hallowed beet has the potential to radically transform health and save lives.

Chapter One

The Beeting Heart

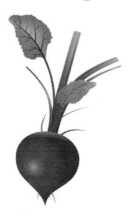

Ancient History

There has been a long and seemingly romantic relationship between humans and beets. It began with the ancestor of all cultivated beets, the wild sea beet, whose leaves have been consumed since prehistoric times. In fact, beetroot was originally grown for its leaves and stems. Beets were first cultivated by ancient Greeks, Romans and Jews who consumed the leaves, but the Romans were the first to enjoy the root originally as a medicine for fevers and other conditions. However, the beet would not become a famous "root" vegetable until the 16th century.

Ancient Aphrodisiac

Beets are a fascinating part of Greek and Roman Mythology. It appears the goddess of beauty and love, Aphrodite (or Venus), attributed her romantic power to the beetroot. The term "aphrodisiac" persists as a tribute to this ostensive beet-goddess. This likely explains why beetroot is portrayed in erotic paintings on brothel walls (the "Lupanar") of ancient Pompeii. It was the aphrodisiac benefit that drove the sun god Apollo and his worshippers to fervently seek out the beetroot. The Greeks presented the beet as an offering to Apollo in the temple at Delphi - the site where Apollo was told by the Oracle that the radish is worth its weight in lead but the beet its weight in silver - second only to horseradish, which was worth its weight in gold.

The heart-shape of the beetroot and leaf and the passionately red color imply a deep connection to the icon of love, the heart. The beet even "bleeds" red. And if the root is the heart then the leaves are the embodiment of its extension, pulsing red through the main "artery" and its smaller "capillaries" which are visibly traceable on a beet leaf. Although there are white beets that exude sugar juice instead of "blood", it is the beet's penetrating red color that creates the drama for what the ancients believed was the essence of its power.

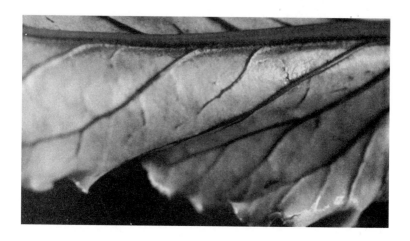

Other historical beet links include:

- Ancient murals portray Romans drinking glasses of what appears to be red wine, but some historians suggest that it is actually beetroot juice.

- In Greek history, Aristotle (384-322 BC) left descriptions about beets, as did his students, noting the depth of red color.

- Beets appear in broths and salads in a cookbook entitled *Apicius*: *The Roman Cookery Book* which was translated in 1958 (Flowers and Rosenbaum) from a compilation of early medicinal and culinary recipes dating back to the first century AD in Tiberius.

- Hippocrates (c 460- 370 BC) the ancient Greek physician and "Father of Medicine" recommended beets for binding wounds, blood cleansing and digestive problems.

- An Assyrian text (800 BC) describes beets growing in the Hanging Gardens of Babylon, one of the wonders of the ancient world.

- In beet folklore, falling in love was considered the consequence of a couple eating from the same beetroot.

- As recent as the early 20th century "taking favors in the beetroot fields" was a popular euphemism for prostitution.

- "Blood Turnip" was once a common name for the garden beet.

- Eating beetroot with garlic will nullify "garlic breath".

- The water left behind from boiled beets was massaged into the scalp nightly as an effective cure for dandruff.

- In 1975 cosmonauts from the USSR welcomed the Apollo 18 astronauts by preparing beetroot soup (borscht) at zero gravity.

- Beetroot can be made into a wine that tastes similar to port.

- Deep red beet juice is used to alleviate hangovers.

More Recent History

The ancients saw mystical qualities in the tender, sweet, earthy beet and ensured its cultivation for the benefit of posterity. From its Mediterranean origins, the beet spread across the Old World through trade route. By the middle ages it was grown for the root and medieval herbalists were hailing its benefits. Beets could be found thriving as a winter vegetable in the monastery gardens of Italy, France and Spain. New edible beetroot varieties were being developed and introduced to northern Europe. At that time, the beet roots were a bit longer and thinner than the modern beet.

The familiar heart-shaped root came in the 16th century and over a few hundred years, became a mainstay in Central and Eastern European cuisine. In England, the beet was also gaining acceptance and by the 19th century it could be found in soup, salad, pudding and desserts. European settlers brought the beet to America and colonial Americans greatly relied upon it for survival during the winter months.

Eventually, it was discovered that beets provided a concentrated source of sugar and an alternative to sugar cane. This eventually led to the emergence of distinctly sweeter varieties such as the "sugar beet" and along with it, sugar factories.

Benevolent Beets

Beets were used throughout history from providing the color in dyes, food coloring, lipstick and rouge to the substrate for fermentation in food and drink that became cultural staples consumed as the "elixir of life". To this day, many people are familiar with the beloved, traditional beet soup called borsch which remains ever-popular in Russia and Eastern Europe.

Currently, there are many varieties of cultivated Beta vulgaris including the leaf vegetables, chard and spinach beet, as well as the root vegetables. Beetroot varieties differ in their shape, size and color. The root color can range from yellow to red with variegated types that resemble candy-stripes. The white-rooted "sugar beet" is used for the production of table sugar (sucrose) and has been cultivated over time to contain up to 20% sugar content. Another beet called mangelwurzel is grown for fodder or animal feed and is too coarse for human consumption. The most familiar one, however, is the intensely red beetroot – the favorite on the radar of health-conscious people these days.

And for good reason…

References for Chapter 1

1. Caballero B, et al. Encyclopedia of Human Nutrition. 2005
2. http://en.wikipedia.org/wiki/Beet
3. http://en.wikipedia.org/wiki/Beetroot
4. http://www.stephennottingham.co.uk/beetroot.htm
5. http://academics.hamilton.edu/foodforthought/Our_Research_files/beet. pdf
6. Beets Varieties, from Heirloom Seedsmen, a website of the Baker Creek Heirloom Seed Company
7. http://rareseeds.com/vegetablesa-c/beetroot.html?gclid=CJSu1pidzLMCF XCmPAoddjMAYA

Chapter Two

The Beetiful Color

The beetroot is a treasure trove of densely-packed, priceless nutrients that the next few chapters will explore. Beets are a member of the Chenopod family and its relatives are (Swiss) chard, spinach and quinoa. These foods have related nutritional value that is not available from other food families. Chenopod phytonutrients continue to show an increasing number of unique health benefits.

Beet nutrition begins with its unrivaled antioxidant pigments found in the root and the green tops as well. The beet's root color is a complex mixture of nitrogen-containing, water-soluble pigments called **beta**lains (bā'tă-lāns). The term derives from **Beta** vulgaris. Betalains are different, however, than the abundant red pigments (anthocyanins) of many fruits and vegetables such as red cabbage, grapes, cherries and plums.

It is the betalains that determine the root color of beets which can range from yellow to a deep red-violet. Collectively, the red to purple-violet betalains are called *betacyanins* (principally betanin), while the yellow to orange pigments are called the *betaxanthins* (principally vulgaxanthin and indicaxanthin). Betanin is the easiest one to remember, as it is the primary pigment in red beets and the best-studied betalain to date. All beets contain the yellow pigments - they are just masked in red beets. Betalains are concentrated in the beet cell and will easily leak out or "bleed" from the beetroot when it is cut or heated.

Antioxidant - Anti-inflammatory

Beet betalains are potent antioxidants. Antioxidants are important because they snuff out or neutralize free radicals, or oxidants, which can be thought of as infinitesimally small yet highly-reactive sparks that cause damage to the body's cells and their DNA. Many types of health problems are associated with an over-abundance of these "radicals" which are "free" to cause excess oxidation with resulting inflammation (oxidative stress). Free radicals are naturally created in the body through metabolism and are taken into the body from the environment and a poor diet. A certain amount of free radical activity is absolutely necessary, but far too often the balance of oxidants versus antioxidants is weighted to the oxidant side. In defense, the body responds by making more of its own antioxidants such as glutathione but is complemented by antioxidants in the diet to protect against free radical injury and maintain an ideal inflammatory balance.

It has not gone unnoticed that betalains have high antioxidant activity which means they act as anti-inflammatory molecules. There are a significant number of well-designed studies to support their role as antioxidants. Betalains have demonstrated 3 to 4 times greater antioxidant activity than vitamin C and some polyphenols such as rutin and catechin. Betanin was shown to reduce free radical damage to fats (lipid peroxidation) and also quiet down enzymes in the body that ignite inflammation (COX-1 and COX-2). Recently published results indicate that the antioxidant capacity of betanin inhibited free radical damage in neutrophils (PMNs). This is important because neutrophils are key white blood cells in the body's inflammatory response.

Antioxidants reduce oxidative stress and inflammation linked to heart disease. It is one mechanism by which beets may offer protection against coronary heart disease and stroke. Several other mechanisms will be discussed in the chapters to come. The beneficial effects demonstrated in beet studies are likely due to multiple components in beets. But as fundamental agents for reducing the risk of chronic diseases, the antioxidants in beets are core. For example, in one lipid study, betalains in beets prevented high total serum cholesterol and high liver triglycerides in rats fed a diet designed to cause both (dyslipidemia). Abnormal fats are linked to blood vessel plaque (atherosclerosis) and other negative metabolic changes such as elevated blood sugar and liver enzymes. Betalains also protect LDL cholesterol from dangerous modifications that contribute to atherosclerosis.

Detoxification

Beets have historically been used for detoxification to cleanse or rid the body of excess toxins. Betalains, particularly betanin, are powerful stimulators of the body's own (phase 2) detoxification enzymes that neutralize free radicals and help clear the system of environmental toxins known as xenobiotics - chemicals foreign to living organisms. This is crucial because there are enormous amounts of chemicals released into the environment yearly. According to a U.S. Cancer Panel, it is estimated that globally, people commonly encounter as many as 80,000 different pollutants daily. Cancer statistics are correlated with environmental toxin exposure. Beets may support the ability of cells to actively neutralize toxins in preventing damage linked to disease risk.

Anti-Cancer

It appears that betanin is an important contributor to the anti-cancer effects of beetroot. In cancer prevention studies, betanin was effective in suppressing the development of multi-organ tumors in experimental animals. Betanin was then tested for its destructive effects (cytotoxic) in androgen-independent human prostate cancer cells (PC-3) and in the well-established estrogen receptor-positive human breast cancer cells (MCF-7). The beetroot extract exhibited a dose-dependent cytotoxic effect in both cancer cell lines tested. Additionally, beet studies also demonstrated that the extract inhibited the growth of other tumor cell lines from the colon, stomach, central nervous system, skin and lungs. Still other studies show that betalains can protect from radiation exposure by increasing the activity of the body's own antioxidant enzymes (superoxide dismutase and glutathione peroxidases) in organs such as liver, spleen and kidney.

Thus, betalain pigments from red beets are invigorating, life-enhancing, protective substances that provide antioxidant, anti-inflammatory, detoxification and anti-cancer benefits. Fortunately, beets just happen to be the best and most importance source of betalains!

Polyphenols – Cellular Rejuvenation

Current evidence for the protective effects of plant nutrients against disease has generated much excitement and created new expectations for bolstering health. It appears that the properties of polyphenols for example, go far beyond their widely-studied antioxidant action. Beets are a rich source of health-promoting polyphenols and carotenoids including luteolin, quercitin, lutein, zeaxanthin and beta-carotene.

Safe Colorant

It is worth mentioning that betalains are useful in the food industry as colorants. The public has shown an increasing preference for natural food colorants rather than synthetic ones in foods, cosmetics, and pharmaceuticals. Betanin, as E162, is used for flavor and color in dairy products, meats, tomato paste, sauces, desserts and breakfast cereals. Betanin appears to be a sensible food additive that not only contributes health benefits, but it has virtually no potential to provoke allergy.

"In the Pink" - Beeturia

Sometimes colorful urine (or stool) is a noticeable side effect from eating beetroot. Producing pink-red urine is distressing because it can be mistaken for blood. It is actually excreted betalain pigments causing the red color. It has been long known, even in folklore, that some individuals excrete red urine after eating beets while others do not. Many investigations have been conducted to determine why some people experience this but without definite conclusions. It has been suggested that beeturia may be linked to food allergies, malabsorption and gut permeability syndromes, genetic factors (polymorphisms) or iron metabolism issues. But even in repeat studies, the same individual may show variation in reproducibility of results. Furthermore, it may be that some people just excrete too little pigment to be noticed. A well-designed study supported this in which urine samples from 100 subjects who ingested 60 mg of beetroot pigment all showed small amounts of pigment in the urine, however, in some participants the concentrations were just too low to appear red. To complicate the matter, the type of beetroot consumed was shown to influence the outcome. Some susceptible people who showed intense urine coloration with one beet variety gave virtually normal urine with another.

The pH of urine affects the color of the pigments. They are stable between pH 4 to 5 but lose their color in alkaline conditions and decompose in acid conditions going from red to yellow. Therefore, if pigment is present in the urine, the color intensity is dependent upon the urinary pH. The human stomach has an average acidity of about pH 2 and in these conditions the beet pigment rapidly decomposes. If this was the major determinant of beeturia, then the occurrence of beeturia would likely be more common in conditions of low stomach acid. This hypothesis was supported by a report of an elderly man who had never displayed beeturia until he began taking an acid-reducing drug for acid (esophageal) reflux. Additionally, the beetroot pigments lose their color in the presence of iron (ferric ions) from the diet. Still other studies report that vitamin C and oxalic acid found in beetroot may protect the pigments from breakdown in the stomach. Investigations into this phenomenon will likely continue but at present it appears that beeturia is dependent upon a person's physiology in regulating the pH of his or her system.

References for Chapter 2

Francis FJ. (1999). *Colorants*. Egan Press. ISBN 1-891127-00-4
Pavokovic D, Krsnik-Rasol M. Food Technol Biotechnol.
  2011;49(2):145-155
Wroblewska M, et al. Lipids Health Dis. 2011;10:178
Zielinska-Przyjemska M, et al. Phytother Res. 2012;26(6):845-52
Zielinska-Przyjemska M, et al. Phytother Res. 2009;23(1):49-55
Kanner J, et al. J Agric Food Chem. 2001;49:5178-85
Kapadia GJ, et al. Cancer Lett. 1996;100:211-14
Kapadia GJ, et al. Anticancer Agents Med Chem. 2011;11(3):280-4
Kapadia GJ, et al. Pharmacol Res. 2003;47(2):141-8
Lu X, et al. Eur J Pharmacol. 2009;615(1-3):223-7
Wettasinghe M, et al. J Agric Food Chem. 2002;50:6704-09
Pedreno MA, et al. J Biol Educ 2000;35:49-51
Lee CS, et al. Nutr Cancer. 2005;53:91-103
Georgiev VG, et al. Plant Foods Hum Nutr. 2010;65(2):105-11
Reddy MK, et al. J Agric Food Chem. 2005;53(23):9268-73
Mitchell SC. Drug Metab Dispos. 2001;29:539-43
Gonzales CA. Br J Nutr. 2006;96:S42-45
Agarwal M, et al. Fitoterapia. 2006;77:91-93
Vali L, et al. Nutrition. 2007;23(2):172-8
http://www.washingtonpost.com/wp-dyn/content/article/2010/05/06/
  AR2010050603813.html
http://en.wikipedia.org/wiki/Betanin
http://en.wikipedia.org/wiki/Beet
www.whfoods.com
http://academics.hamilton.edu/foodforthought/Our_Research_files/beet.pdf

Chapter Three

A Beet More

Betaine

There are more jewels in the beet treasury that contribute to its superfood status. Another "beta" compound, distinctly different from betalains, was discovered in beet juice and was named betaine. Its role is to regulate the water content (osmosis) in the beet cell. For the science-lovers, betaine is the simple amino acid glycine with 3 attached methyl groups (tri-methyl-glycine). Donating these vital methyl groups to needy human biochemistry has helped betaine earns its place as a valued nutrient.

Methyl is Magical

In human health, betaine protects cells, proteins and enzymes from environmental stress such as low water (dehydration), excess salt or extreme temperature. Betaine is also used in cosmetics and beauty supplies for its water-holding (humectant) effect. As a methyl donor, betaine reduces dangerous levels of an amino acid called homocysteine. A high blood homocysteine level is a risk factor for heart disease due to its damaging effects in the blood vessels. Betaine donates a methyl group to homocysteine converting it to methionine to form S-adenosyl-methionine (SAMe). This step is critically important because it ensures the continuing process of methylation which, in addition to cardiovascular health, is vital to proper prenatal development, mental health (particularly mood), cancer prevention, detoxification, immune function, inflammatory balance and the health of other organs.

In a large cross-sectional survey (ATTICA study), betaine intake led to decreases in homocysteine plus two additional markers of inflammation: C-reactive protein and tumor necrosis factor.

Studies show that betaine protects the liver and may be a promising treatment for nonalcoholic fatty liver disease as well as alcohol-induced liver damage. It promotes liver cell regeneration and reduces high liver triglycerides. Multiple mechanisms contribute to betaine's beneficial liver effects such as antioxidant, methyl donor, mitochondrial support and prevention of excess liver fat (lipotropic). Betaine stimulates the liver to keep bile flowing freely through the bile ducts. This safeguards the condition of the liver and gallbladder, contributing to peak digestion and the elimination of toxins.

Athletic Actions

Yet another feature of betaine is the power-boost it lends to athletic performance. Several recent studies performed at different U.S. colleges reported evidence of improved aerobic and anaerobic metabolism including gains in muscle strength plus the quantity and quality of repetitions. Researchers speculate that betaine may raise creatine levels, lower lactic acid levels and/or support growth hormone production in the body as possible mechanisms for the increased muscle strength. Although these studies were conducted with betaine as a pure supplement, here's the point: beets contain betaine which may be a contributing factor to what you are about to read in the next chapters regarding beet consumption and enhanced athletic performance.

Betaine is just another instrument in the beet symphony that in concert produces a crescendo of improved function and disease prevention.

Folate

Methyl & More

Beets are rich in another methyl donor - folate (aka folic acid). Like betaine, folate helps lower blood levels of homocysteine and raise SAMe levels. Studies show that both SAMe and folate are effective for reducing the symptoms of depression. With regard to depression, it must be mentioned here that beets also contain tryptophan. This is the amino acid that builds serotonin in the body. Serotonin is well known for its importance in proper mood, sleep, sexuality and appetite. Low levels of tryptophan are seen in depressed patients and correlate with the degree of depression. There is a growing campaign for non-pharmaceutical alternatives in treating depression disorders. Hopefully, consuming more beets rich in folate, betaine and tryptophan will help meet this widespread need. Moreover, folate is necessary for healthy gums, blood cell formation, the prevention of birth defects and multiple functions of the gastrointestinal, immune and cardiovascular systems.

Boron

The beet is a very boron-dependent crop which makes it a rich source of this trace mineral. Farmers know that a lack of boron will cause the new beet shoots to deteriorate. The importance of boron to human health was just recently uncovered in the 1980's.

You may recall in chapter one, that the aphrodisiac or sexually-invigorating property of beets was first described by the early Greeks and Romans. It is now scientifically demonstrated that there is a basis to the aphrodisiac claims. Evidence points to the abundance of boron as a key factor. In human and animal studies boron is shown to increase steroid hormones, particularly estrogen and testosterone. Additionally, boron is shown to reduce the loss of vitamin D, calcium and magnesium from the body. For these reasons combined, it is best known in healthcare for improving bones and easing the symptoms and incidence of arthritis.

Nutrient Density

Beets also contain more familiar nutrients. Besides folate, the dominant vitamins in beets appear to be vitamins A and C, along with vitamin K and the B vitamins. In addition to boron, the dominant minerals present as potassium, calcium, magnesium, manganese and phosphorus, but beets also contain iron, zinc, copper, sodium and selenium. Potassium is particularly beneficial for cardiovascular health. Beets contain respectable levels of insoluble and soluble fiber and contain phytosterols, both of which have been studied for their beneficial effects on metabolism and the digestive tract. Nutritionally, fresh beets and beet root juice retain their nutrient content better than canned and processed beets.

Beets contain simple carbohydrates lending natural sweetness, but beets are also very nutrient-dense which qualifies them as a sensible energy fuel source. This, of course, is not the case with refined and processed carbohydrates which are linked to many health problems. Beets deliver about 2 grams of protein per serving (4 oz) and have a very low fat content.

It is essential to note that sources for beet nutritional facts are not consistent. It is not entirely accurate to list the weight or percentage of each nutrient due to conflicting data sources and beet conditions (i.e. cooked vs. raw, variety, stored vs. fresh). The geographical area where beets are grown can make all the difference in the nutritional profile. Key factors such as soil richness, year-to-year changes in temperature, sunlight, rainfall and fertilizers, in addition to the effects of shipping and storage, all influence the nutrient content of vegetables such as beets. Organically grown vegetables show significant differences from conventionally grown produce in nutritional data. Pesticide residue should be also taken into account, as these chemicals result in detoxification burdens for the body.

Anti-Aging

The beetroot is overflowing with antioxidant-rich betalains. It is high in betaine, boron and folate which increase its nutrient density. It has all the extra supporting nutrients and endearing history of a real superfood. It outshines in clinical studies and looks to be the apparent remedy for all that ails. Add up these descriptions and the definition of the perfect anti-aging food *almost* surfaces; *almost* because there is one more factor in this rousing root that will forever change the human-beet relationship. With abundantly accumulating research, this next beet nutrient should put beets and beet products back on every table.

And just a note: Some people may be concerned that beets also contain oxalic acid (less than 1%) which is a universal component of plants for mineral (i.e. calcium) binding and protection from herbivores. Oxalic acid is broken down during cooking. Eating too much oxalic acid (i.e. approx. 16 cups of raw spinach) can be detrimental because it can bind dietary calcium and make it unavailable for absorption. Most people do not consume enough oxalic acid in vegetables, or for long enough, to negatively affect calcium absorption.

The following chapters mark a new history for the bodacious beet - one of not only enhancing, but of saving lives.

References for Chapter 3

Craig SA. Am J Clin Nutr. 2004;80(3):539-49
Kharbanda KK, et al. Int J Hepatol. 2012;2012:962183. Epub 2011 Dec 8
Kharbanda KK. Semin Liver Dis. 2009;29(2):155-65
Barak AJ, et al. Alcohol. 1996;13:395-398
Barak AJ, et al. Alcohol Clin Exp Res. 1993;17:552-555
Murakami T, et al. J Nutr Sci Vitaminol. 1998;44:249-25
Sandeep M. World J Gastroenterol. 2011;17(32):3663-64
Papakostas GI, et al. Can J Psychiatry. 2012;57(7):406-13
Bottiglieri T, et al. Drugs. 1994;48(2):137-52
Bressa GM. Acta Neurol Scand Suppl. 1994;154:7-14
Papakostas GI, et al. Am J Psychiatry. 2010;167(8):942-8
Lord R, et al. Lab Eval Integ Func Med. 2008, (boron p.11 / tryptophan p.220-1)
http://www.nal.usda.gov/afsic/pubs/srb0003.shtml
Hoffman JR, et al. J Int Soc Sports Nutr. 2009;6:7
Armstrong LE, et al. J Strength Cond Res. 2008;22(3):851-60
Lee EC, et al. J IntSoc Sports Nutr. 2010;7:27
Detopoulou P, et al. Am J Clin Nutr. 2008;87(2):424-30
http://en.wikipedia.org/wiki/Beetroot

Chapter Four

The Unbeetable Benefit

Miracle Molecule

Health-conscious people rarely disdain beets; those that do may be reconsidering at this point. Any memories of canned beets being force-fed to children need to be purged. Considering America's current state of health, there is no time like the present to start eating beets and drinking beet root juice.

Arguably, the most valuable contribution that beets make to modern wellbeing comes from a surprising newcomer. Long known as a nutrient for plants, the inorganic **nitrate** content of beetroot makes it one of the best concentrated sources. When ingested, nitrate is reduced to **nitrite** which then becomes the molecular powerhouse called **nitric oxide** or **N-O**. It is referred to as a "miracle" molecule and the faithful beet delivers the nitrate for N-O power. The astounding effects of N-O have also caught the attention of athletes and clinicians. Beet sales are way up and so is the bar for competing superfoods.

Building N-O in the body through beet root nitrate *is* the unbeatable benefit of beets. In fact, the beet's root is considered the "super-root" because of its ability to uptake and concentrate high levels of nitrate from the soil. Improving the level of N-O in the body can prevent, slow and even reverse many health problems particularly, cardiovascular disease. N-O is first and foremost a signaling molecule that influences critical biological functions by sending messages or "signals" to cells. It is the subject of over 130,000 published scientific papers and even has a medical journal called *Nitric Oxide* devoted solely to the understanding of its protective role in human health and disease.

The signaling properties of N-O were discovered in the 1980's by 3 scientists who later were awarded the Nobel Prize in Medicine in 1998. The central feature of a number of chronic disorders, especially heart disease, is the inability to make or respond to N-O. Therefore, the discovery of N-O represents an extremely important advance in science and medicine for the treatment of disease in general. N-O is the master of regulation and controls blood flow to every organ and tissue. If it is not adequately available to perform its many roles, then the body starts to fail on every level.

Safety of Nitrates and Nitrites

The production of N-O from beets starts with nitrate and nitrite. But before that process is explained, it is important to understand more about them. These two "good guys" have had their reputations undeservingly pulled into question and sadly this led to years of misunderstanding regarding their significance.

Nitrate (NO_3^-) and nitrite (NO_2^-) belong to a family of compounds that contain the elements, nitrogen and oxygen. They are released into soil and water from dead and decaying organic matter and fertilizers. The plants use nitrate to build protein. Eating the plants as fruits and vegetables delivers nitrates into the body. Another source of nitrate and nitrite is processed meats such as deli meats, where they are added and used as natural preservatives. In meats, nitrate converts to nitrite as the primary preservative that protects against rancidity (oxidation of fats), controls the growth of bacteria, preserves the flavor and provides the red color (reaction with myoglobin). Lastly, nitrate and nitrite are also produced naturally in the body.

About 80% of the average adult intake of nitrates and nitrites come from eating vegetables. Vegetarians who eat predominantly fresh vegetables and people who eat "heart-friendly" diets undoubtedly consume more nitrates. It is widely-supported in medical literature that diets rich in fruits and vegetables reduce the risk of cardiovascular disease and cancer. It is now known that some of those health benefits are attributable to the nitrates.

In the 1960's, concern arose about the nitrate and nitrite content of foods. They were thought to be a possible cause of cancer due to their potential for nitrosamine formation in rat studies. The (epidemiological) association between high nitrate/nitrite and cancer - if it was found to exist at all - was very weak. Fortunately, continuing studies looked at the long list of "other" meat-related compounds and even meat-related lifestyle factors as carcinogenic suspects.

Though now largely discredited, these ideas led some countries to set limits on the level of nitrates and nitrites in food and water. In the field of science it takes time for new findings to change established viewpoints. In contrast to old concerns, there is now evidence that nitrate and nitrite play a very active and key role both directly and indirectly in supporting wellbeing. Consider the fact that these same nitrates and nitrites are found not only in cured meats but in vegetables, especially the green leafy and colorful varieties which are linked to the *prevention* of cancer. If nitrate and nitrite are carcinogens then vegetables are carcinogenic! In fact, a person eating a vegetable-rich DASH diet (Dietary Approaches to Stop Hypertension), known to reduce high blood pressure and the risk for heart disease, has an intake of nitrates *five times higher* than what the World Health Organization proposes, due to the questionable nitrate concern.

As a final point, one of the most compelling arguments for the requirement of nitrate and nitrite in the diet: the breast milk of newly nursing mothers naturally contains high levels of both with nitrite levels higher than any other food or beverage. These indispensable nutrients are present in mother's milk to ensure growth and development with a strong immune system for the child.

Evidence shows that longstanding concerns about the toxicity of ingested nitrate and nitrite are overstated. In fact, the emerging physiological data on nitrite as an essential nutrient molecule seems analogous to a vitamin. Perhaps the designation "Vitamin N" will eventually be ascribed to this important nutrient that many are lacking.

N-O spells YES!

The high dietary nitrate found in beetroot is the source for the production of nitric oxide. When N-O is created and released in the body, it penetrates cell membranes and sends off crucial signals inside *every* cell, tissue, organ and system. Is this a good thing? Absolutely yes, it gets the blood flowing! For example, N-O commands:

- blood vessels to relax so they can expand which reduces blood pressure and increases circulation and oxygen to cells

- platelets to become less sticky thus preventing abnormal blood clots and blood vessel plaque build-up (atherosclerosis)

- the immune system to destroy invading disease-producing agents and cancer cells

- brain cells to communicate with each other for proper brain function and mood

At least one third of Americans have confirmed high blood pressure (hypertension) and many more do not even know they have it. In the American Heart Association journal, *Hypertension,* researchers showed that drinking 500ml of beetroot juice (approx. 16 oz or 2 cups) lowered blood pressure within an hour. After 3-4 hours, blood pressure was substantially reduced. Furthermore, the pressure lowering effect remained for up to 24 hours after consuming the juice. The drop in blood pressure was matched with peak increases in blood nitrite levels that came from ingesting the beet juice. The beet nitrate was reduced to nitrite and then to N-O. The endothelium (inner lining of blood vessels) used N-O to signal its surrounding smooth muscle to relax. This caused the blood vessels to dilate, reducing pressure and increasing blood flow around the body. This study clearly demonstrated that dietary nitrate contributes to the beneficial effects of beets.

Nitrate to N-O

Just how does the body convert nitrate from beets into life-saving N-O? It is a process that takes a couple of important steps:

- Nitrate from the diet is absorbed in the stomach and small intestine and enters the bloodstream. As blood circulates, the salivary glands pull the nitrate in and concentrate it in saliva. Oral bacteria found in the tongue (crypts) change the nitrate to nitrite. The nitrite is swallowed and in the presence of sufficient stomach acid, much of the nitrite is converted to N-O. This is the goal. [Indeed, use of anti-bacterial mouthwashes and products that kill "germs" in the mouth will blunt or inhibit this important process and there will not be a benefit. Antacids and proton pump inhibitors, that reduce stomach acid, will also interfere with nitrite conversion to N-O.]

- When N-O, which regulates many functions, has done its job, it breaks down. Nitrate is re-produced or "recycled" from the breakdown of N-O. It was once believed that N-O formation could only happen through a pathway that involved the amino acid, L-arginine. It is now known that N-O is broken down forming nitrate again which recycles through nitrite to regenerate more N-O. This is called the *"nitrate→nitrite→N-O pathway"* and is the main pathway for making N-O in people over 40 years old and in reduced oxygen or cellular stress situations. This process is occurring second by second in the blood and various tissues. The discovery of this pathway allowed scientists a greater understanding of how nitrates protect the cardiovascular system in healthy individuals as well as those with heart disease.

Entero-Salivary Circulation of Nitrate from Beets

The major source of nitrate/nitrite in the body comes from vegetable consumption (about 80%), but they are also produced naturally in the body through the metabolism and recycling of N-O.

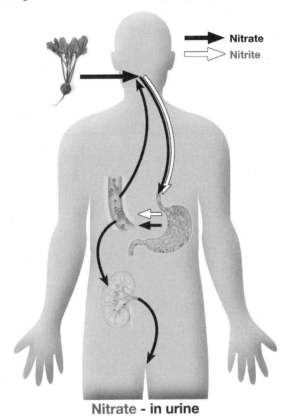

Nitrate - in urine

Beet nitrate is swallowed and enters the blood from the stomach and small intestine. As nitrate circulates, about 25% of it will be taken up by the salivary glands creating saliva that is 10 times more concentrated in nitrate than blood (some nitrate will be lost to urine within 48 hrs). Oral bacteria of the tongue reduce nitrate to nitrite. Nitrite becomes concentrated and is swallowed. The stomach acidity allows for nitrite reduction to N-O. Both nitrite and N-O are taken into the system and become part of the nitrate→nitrite→N-O pathway for increased vasodilation, circulation, oxygen delivery and other signaling functions.

Beets are an amazing source of concentrated nitrate and other heart-healthy nutrients. The following chart shows other foods that are nitrate-rich and will help increase nitrate levels in the body. The role of nitrate and nitrite for improving N-O levels in the body may provide the rationale for "food therapy" using vegetables such as beets in the natural treatment and prevention of cardiovascular disease.

Main fruit/vegetable dietary sources of nitrate

Nitrate Value	Nitrate Content (per kg fresh vegetable)	Common Vegetables
Very High	2500 mg/40 mmol	Beetroot and beetroot juice, lettuce, rocket (arugula), spinach
High	1000-2500 mg/18-40 mmol	Chinese cabbage, endive, leek, parsley, kohlrabi
Moderate	500-1000 mg/9-18 mmol	Cabbage, dill, turnips, carrot juice
Low	200-500 mg/3-9 mmol	Broccoli, carrot, cauliflower, cucumber, pumpkin, V8 vegetable juice,
Very low	<200 mg/< 3 mmol	Asparagus, artichoke, broad beans, green beans, peas, capsicum, tomato, watermelon, tomato, sweet potato, potato, garlic, onion, eggplant, mushroom

The Power of N-O

In younger people, plenty of N-O is made in the endothelium from L-arginine and oxygen. With age and especially with poor health habits, the endothelium becomes less efficient at producing N-O. It will eventually lose the ability to produce any N-O. This is called "endothelial dysfunction". In fact, loss of N-O with age is the hallmark of atherosclerosis which is the disease that develops from endothelial dysfunction. In atherosclerosis, plaque builds up inside the arteries and other blood vessels interfering with the ability to carry oxygen-rich blood around the body. It leads to heart attacks and strokes and is the number one cause of death in the developed world.

That is why the body provides a perfect back-up plan for N-O production using nitrate. It may help to think of nitrate as a critical storage form of N-O. It can convert to N-O anywhere when the body needs it. With age and with less oxygen, there is greater dependence on the nitrate→nitrite→N-O pathway. N-O derived from nitrite has been shown to prevent cell injury in situations where oxygen is inadequate resulting in free radical damage to tissues (ischemic injury).

Nitrate and nitrite production of N-O from beets can benefit the following conditions which are known to be linked to low N-O. In each of the follow conditions, it will help to:

- Arthritis - increase circulation and decrease nerve irritation and inflammation in joints associated with arthritis pain

- Altitude Sickness – increase circulation and oxygen availability

- Asthma - widen "hyper-responsive" airways, calming the immune reaction and relaxing muscles and nerves

- Bladder problems – remediate incontinence and infections

- Cancer - support treatment by increasing blood flow and oxygen around the tumor, sensitize cancer cells to radiation, limit DNA damage from radiation and boost cancer-killing ability of immune cells

- COPD (chronic obstructive pulmonary disease) - improve lung function and ease breathlessness

- Cognitive function - increase brain cell communication to help prevent dementia and Alzheimer's disease

- Diabetes (type 2) – support insulin function which helps prevent insulin resistance and the circulation-destroying complications that result from it

- Erectile Dysfunction (ED) – relieve ED as it is actually a circulation problem and an early warning sign of cardiovascular disease

- Eye Disease – increase ocular blood flow and relieve intraocular pressure (glaucoma)

- Infections – support the immune system in destroying invading micro-organisms

- Insomnia – maintain deep or "recovery sleep" (REM) especially with aging

- Kidney Disease – regulate blood flow to kidneys, excretion of sodium and govern filtration rate

- Mood/Depression – support mood as levels of N-O are significantly lower in depression vs. non-depression

- Memory Loss – increase cerebral blood flow for short and long-term memory

- Osteoporosis – regulate bone remodeling

- Overweight – increase glucose uptake through insulin signaling (Glut4 transport) and reduce the risk of heart disease in obesity

- Stomach ulcers – heal ulcers, protect stomach mucosal lining and inhibit bacterial overgrowth

- Stress – relieve "stress-induced" behavior

- Skin Disease – contribute to barrier-function, support the healing process and protect keratinocytes from UV radiation

- Tardive dyskinesia – act as a therapeutic option for treatment

- Sickle cell anemia – improve circulation

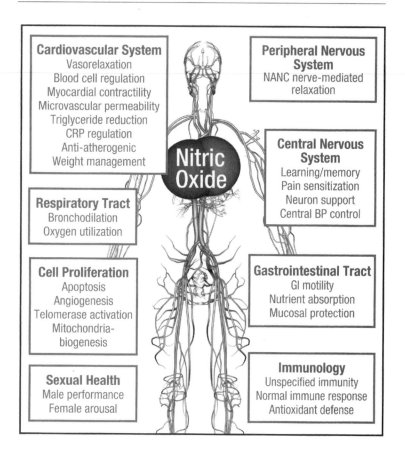

Cardiovascular System
Vasorelaxation
Blood cell regulation
Myocardial contractility
Microvascular permeability
Triglyceride reduction
CRP regulation
Anti-atherogenic
Weight management

Peripheral Nervous System
NANC nerve-mediated relaxation

Nitric Oxide

Central Nervous System
Learning/memory
Pain sensitization
Neuron support
Central BP control

Respiratory Tract
Bronchodilation
Oxygen utilization

Cell Proliferation
Apoptosis
Angiogenesis
Telomerase activation
Mitochondria-
biogenesis

Gastrointestinal Tract
GI motility
Nutrient absorption
Mucosal protection

Sexual Health
Male performance
Female arousal

Immunology
Unspecified immunity
Normal immune response
Antioxidant defense

In summary, nitrate and nitrite in beets and other foods can be metabolized to N-O and promote cardiovascular and broad-spectrum benefits. The collective body of evidence suggests that foods containing nitrate and nitrite, particularly beets, provide significant health benefits.

So eat your beets or pick up your glass of beetroot juice and drink-up. Salute!

References for Chapter 4

Bryan NS, et al. Free Radic Biol Med. 2008;45(4):468-74
Milkowski A, et al. Nitric Oxide. 2010;22(2):110-9
Webb AJ, et al. Hypertension. 2008;51(3):784-90
Bryan NS, Zand J. The Nitric Oxide Solution. Austin: Neogenis. 2010
http://www.cdc.gov/mmwr/preview/mmwrhtml/su6001a21.htm
    (hypertension)
Hord NG. Curr Atheroscler Rep. 2011;13(6):484-92
Machha A, Schechter AN. Eur J Nutr. 2011;50(5):293-303
Machha A, Schechter AN. Nutr Rev. 2012;70(6):367-72
Lefer DJ. Arch Pharm Res. 2009;32(8):1127-38
Hord NG, et al. Am J Clin Nutr. 2009;90:1-10
Kolluru GK, et al. Circulation. 2012;126(16):1939-1940
Shiva S, et al. Basic Res Cardiol. 2009;144(2):113-9
Murillo D, et al. Nitric Oxide. 2011;25(2):70-80
Tang Y, et al. Curr Opin Lipidol. 2011;22(1):11-15
Garg HK, Bryan NS. Kidney Int. 2009;75(11):1140-4
Qin L, et al. Proc Natl Acad Sci USA. 2012;109(33):13434-9

Chapter Five

Go Beetroot!

Beets and Performance

Along the trail of beet benefits, the highlights have been the betalain pigments and other plant nutrients, betaine, vitamins, minerals, fiber and in particular, the high concentration of natural nitrate. As the precursor for N-O production, nitrate helps to widen the blood vessels causing an increase in circulation and oxygen delivery to all cells. For the elite athlete or anyone who values exercise and an active life, this feature of nitrate is critical. Nitrate contributes to the physiology of performance, which is the focus of this chapter.

2 Pathways for N-O Generation

The real influence of nitrate from beets occurs after it has been reduced to nitrite and further reduced to N-O. This reaction happens when and where there is a need for N-O in the body.

Thus far, the discussion of N-O has focused on one of two available pathways for N-O production called the nitrate→nitrite→N-O pathway. But to better understand how exercise performance is enhanced, a discussion of the connection to another pathway for N-O production is necessary. Many athletes are perhaps more familiar with this pathway called the L-arginine pathway. It does not use nitrate for N-O production, but rather enzymes such as endothelial nitric oxide synthase (eNOS) and an amino acid called L-arginine (plus oxygen and cofactors).

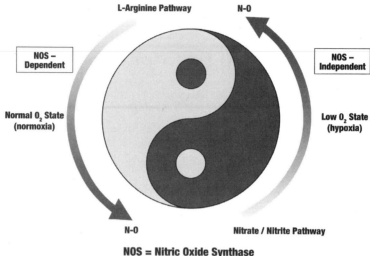

L-Arginine Pathway   N-O

NOS – Dependent

NOS – Independent

Normal O$_2$ State (normoxia)

Low O$_2$ State (hypoxia)

N-O   Nitrate / Nitrite Pathway

NOS = Nitric Oxide Synthase

As previously mentioned, N-O sends a signal to the blood vessel smooth muscles for relaxation. In the L-arginine pathway, the NOS enzymes in the endothelium (eNOS) make N-O from L-arginine. In physical exercise, the eNOS enzymes can be stimulated to make more N-O when blood is rushing against the endothelium as a result of the acute increase in blood flow and blood pressure caused by exercise (sheer stress). This process turns up the volume for more N-O by the eNOS enzymes which in turn relaxes the vessels and keeps blood pressure down. This process keeps the blood vessels supple and healthy.

Now for the connection: when physical activity increases the demand for N-O, the body may need more than can be made by the eNOS enzymes in the blood vessels. If the delivery of blood to the muscles and other tissues cannot keep up with the demands of exercise, the tissues may be briefly starved of oxygen (and other nutrients delivered by the blood).

This is where nitrite, created from the nitrate in beets, comes to the rescue for the athlete. In areas of the body that have low oxygen, the conversion of nitrite to N-O becomes very efficient. It is essential to have available nitrate because the eNOS enzyme does NOT work well without oxygen. The message here is that nitrate and nitrite help the body make more N-O in states of reduced oxygen. This keeps the blood vessels open and the blood flowing under conditions where eNOS cannot. [This is the reason that the nitrate to N-O pathway is so important with age – the aging endothelium becomes dysfunctional and cannot make N-O through eNOS and L-arginine. The resulting endothelial dysfunction leads to hypertension and atherosclerosis which further worsen the ability to make N-O by eNOS in a vicious cycle. The inability to use L-arginine and eNOS begins to happen after age 40 years and for that reason, nitrate-rich foods like beets become imperative as a source for N-O]. So while we have two systems to make N-O in the body, only the system fueled by dietary nitrate can ensure the production of N-O in advancing age and under stressed states such as intense exercise.

Nitrate serves the performance-driven athlete in several other ways:

In addition to increasing circulation, beet nitrate through N-O acts to reduce the amount of oxygen needed by muscles in physical activity. One of the most amazing benefits of increased nitrate production of N-O is found in the cell's own energy factory – the mitochondria. The body creates energy as ATP (adenosine triphosphate) in these tiny organelles of the cell. N-O's influence is to not only increase the number of mitochondria, but also their efficiency of energy production.

There are now more mitochondria making more energy to support exercise over time. This is a profound effect because the N-O produced from nitrate can:

1. increase the potential for energy production

2. lower the amount of oxygen needed by muscles in physical activity to produce energy as ATP (or lowers the oxygen cost of exercise)

3. reduce the amount of ATP energy needed to cause muscles to contract

The 3 mechanisms above, together with the enhancement of blood flow, add up to powerful ways beets and beet root juice can enhance performance.

Here is a simple "bi-directional" link between N-O and exercise that might be easier to remember:

- Exercise improves the ability to produce N-O

- N-O improves the ability to exercise

The increase in mitochondrial efficiency appears to be due to the improvement in oxidative phosphorylation efficiency (P/O ratio). The whole cell can benefit from this improved mitochondrial efficiency which reflects the state of a person's health. In fact, it has been stated that all theories of aging are really secondary to one unifying theory that aging is decreased energy production by the mitochondria.

Recent studies have shown that drinking beet root juice daily or as a single dose before exercise is linked to this enhanced "exercise economy" which means it costs less oxygen to exercise – a kind of fuel economy. In the best of these studies, the use of nitrate-rich beet juice was compared to nitrate-depleted beet juice as a placebo. This nitrate-depleted beet juice enabled scientists to show, for the first time, that nitrate is the active ingredient underlying the exercise benefits.

Beet N-O Potential

There is much discussion among researchers about the best methods for measuring N-O. It is very important to look for beets and beet products that have had their nitric oxide production potential measured. This currently is performed by two complementary methods. High performance liquid chromatography (HPLC) is one sensitive and selective method for accurately determining nitrite and nitrate content. Vegetables, including beets, are primarily rich in nitrate with much less nitrite. In the body, only about 5% of dietary nitrate is metabolized to nitrite with a mere portion of the nitrite being further metabolized to N-O. HPLC testing can detect precise amounts of nitrate and nitrite in beets but cannot predict how they will be used to produce N-O. Ozone-Based Chemiluminescence testing is now considered the most accurate, sensitive and widely used N-O detection method. This technique measures N-O, therefore, it can provide evidence that the nitrate and nitrite in beets are actually generating N-O. In order to make a well-informed purchase, consumers should look for products that use both testing methods.

Beet Stamina

There have been several studies noting the positive effects of beet juice on human exercise and performance. In research conducted by Exeter University, published in the journal *Medicine and Science in Sports and Exercise*, scientists found cyclists who drank 500 ml. of beetroot juice several hours before their ride were able to cycle up to 20% longer than those who drank a placebo nitrate-deficient beet juice. The lead author, Professor Andrew Jones, said, "This is the first time we've studied the effects of beetroot juice, and the high nitrate levels found in it, on simulated competition." Other studies by Dr. Jones identified several situations such as cycling and running events in which beet juice increased performance up to 15%.

In one of Dr. Jones's studies summarized above, researchers found that drinking beet juice appeared to boost exercise stamina. Eight men drank 500 ml. of beet juice daily for six consecutive days before undergoing a series of cycling-based fitness tests. Results showed that after drinking the beetroot juice, the subjects were able to cycle for an average of 92 seconds longer as compared to their cycling time after drinking blackcurrant juice for the same amount of time. A side effect observed in these studies was that the participants also had a lower resting blood pressure after drinking the beet juice. This observed effect was attributed to the increased N-O availability caused by the nitrate in beet juice. In an era when cycling and running events are won by fractions of a second, it is easy to understand why beet juice was such a popular pre-event beverage at the London 2012 Olympics!

The following table lists some of the studies that have supported the notion that beet juice can improve exercise performance.

Effects of dietary beet root juice on exercise performance.

Beet form (juice/ whole)	Exercise type	Exercise time in Placebo	Exercise time in Beet	% increase in endurance due to beet juice	p value/ reference	
Beetroot juice, 6 days	Cycling	9:43	11:15	**15.8%**	<0.01	Bailey et al. 2009 94
Beetroot juice, 6 days	Knee extension	9:46	12:14	**25%**	<0.01	Bailey SJ et al. 2010 96
Beetroot juice, 2 days	Arm and leg cycling	8:44	9:23	**7.5%**	0.13	Larsen et al. 2010 95
Beetroot juice, 6 days	Running	7:36	8:42	**15%**	<0.01	Lansley KE et al. 2011a 98
Beetroot juice, single dose	Cycling (time trial)	27:42	26:54	**2.7%**	<0.01	Lansley KE et al. 2011b 101
Beetroot juice, 6 days	Cycling (time trial)	16:05	15:53	**1%**	<0,005	Cermak NM et al. 2012 103

Time of exercise means the total time necessary to reach exhaustion or, in cycling, a specific distance.

References for Chapter 5

Nisoli E, et al. J Cell Sci. 2006;119(Pt 14):2855-62

www.ausport.gov.au/__data/assets/pdf_file/0009/466029/Beetroot_juice_
Nitrate_11-_website_fact_sheet.pdf

Fulford J, et al. J Appl Physiol. 2011;110:591-600

hppt://en.wikipedia.org/wiki/Beetroot

Bailey SJ, et al. J Appl Physiol. 2009;107:1144-55

Bailey SJ, et al. J Appl Physiol. 2010;109:135-48

Lundberg JO, et al. Cardiovasc Res. 2011;89:525-532

Lanskey KE, et al. Med Sci Sports Exerc. 2011;43(6):1125-31

Lanskey KE, et al. J Appl Physiol. 2011;110:591-600

Larsen FJ, et al. Free Radic Biol Med. 2010;48:342-47

Larsen FJ, et al. Cell Metabol. 2011;13(2):149-59

Clementi E, et al. Comp Biochem Physiol A Mol Integr Physiol.
2005;142:102-110

Cermak NM, et al. Int J Sport Nutr Exerc Metab. 2012;22:64–71

Chapter Six

How to Take Control of Your N-O Level to "Beet the Odds"

Choosing the Right Product

By now it is understood that beets are a great source for the nitrate that generates N-O. However, because only about 5% of beet nitrate is metabolized in a process that takes over an hour, serious beet enthusiasts are seeking out concentrated beet products such as beet juice and dried beet powder or crystals. Organic beets are considered the best, but they still show wide variation in their nitrate and nitrite content as tested by HPLC. In fact, consumers should carefully examine a beet product label to verify that testing was performed to measure the nitrate and nitrite content along with the amount of N-O produced as measured by ozone-based chemiluminesence testing. It is the most accurate way to compare potency among products and helps eliminate the pretenders. It is wise to look for a product that adheres to strict specifications for growing conditions such as soil nutrient content and harvest times, and for the drying process because these types of issues affect the nitrate and nitrite content of the beets.

Patent-Pending Nitric Oxide Indicator Strips

Currently, there are no routine clinical or diagnostic tests to measure N-O. However, nitrate and nitrite have been recently

53

shown to be markers for how much N-O the body is producing. This is great news because without a doubt, everyone who is concerned about health or performance should be interested in how much N-O he or she is making.

Fortunately, there is a place to get a simple, inexpensive test for measuring total body N-O status. The test uses a non-invasive indicator strip that measures nitrite in the saliva. These indicator strips provide an indirect way to measure the amount of N-O in the body. This eliminates the guesswork in attempting to enhance N-O levels in health and performance. For example, it would be ideal for people to know what their personal beet root juice requirement is for achieving an optimum N-O level. With these patent-pending indicator strips, this can now be tracked and adjusted.

This is invaluable information for everyone who is trying to stay healthy and prevent medical problems and for the athlete who wants peak performance through increased levels of nitric oxide as a natural performance builder. But of course, testing N-O is particularly appreciated by anyone with an existing medical problem because low N-O has been linked to nearly all health issues. Improving N-O levels has been shown to ameliorate some conditions and slow the progression of others.

The indicator strips are a way to monitor progress. As low N-O underlies cardiovascular and other diseases, it would seem that every patient should be tested for N-O by doctors in clinics. N-O even helps medications and nutritional supplements work better through improved circulation.

According to the research compiled by the company that creates the patent-pending indicator strips, most people over 40 years old are low in N-O. Although younger people generally have an easier time generating sufficient N-O and are expected to show a normal reading on the indicator strip, or at least better than the over 40's, they often compromise their production of N-O through poor eating habits and lifestyle stress.

The fine-tuned athlete, or those trying to become one, will certainly find the strips helpful. This group contributes to the multi-billion dollar sport supplement industry investing in a variety of supplements to boost athletic performance. To be able to verify if those supplements are working to support an increase in N-O would alone make the strips a worthy investment.

This simple but powerful tool can be part of the strategy to improve the N-O levels in the body, giving users the power to monitor their progress and help encourage compliance with diet and especially beet consumption. The site is named nitricoxidediagnostics.com

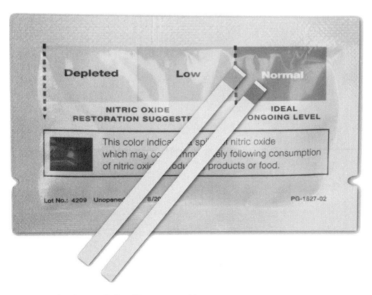

www.nitricoxidediagnostics.com